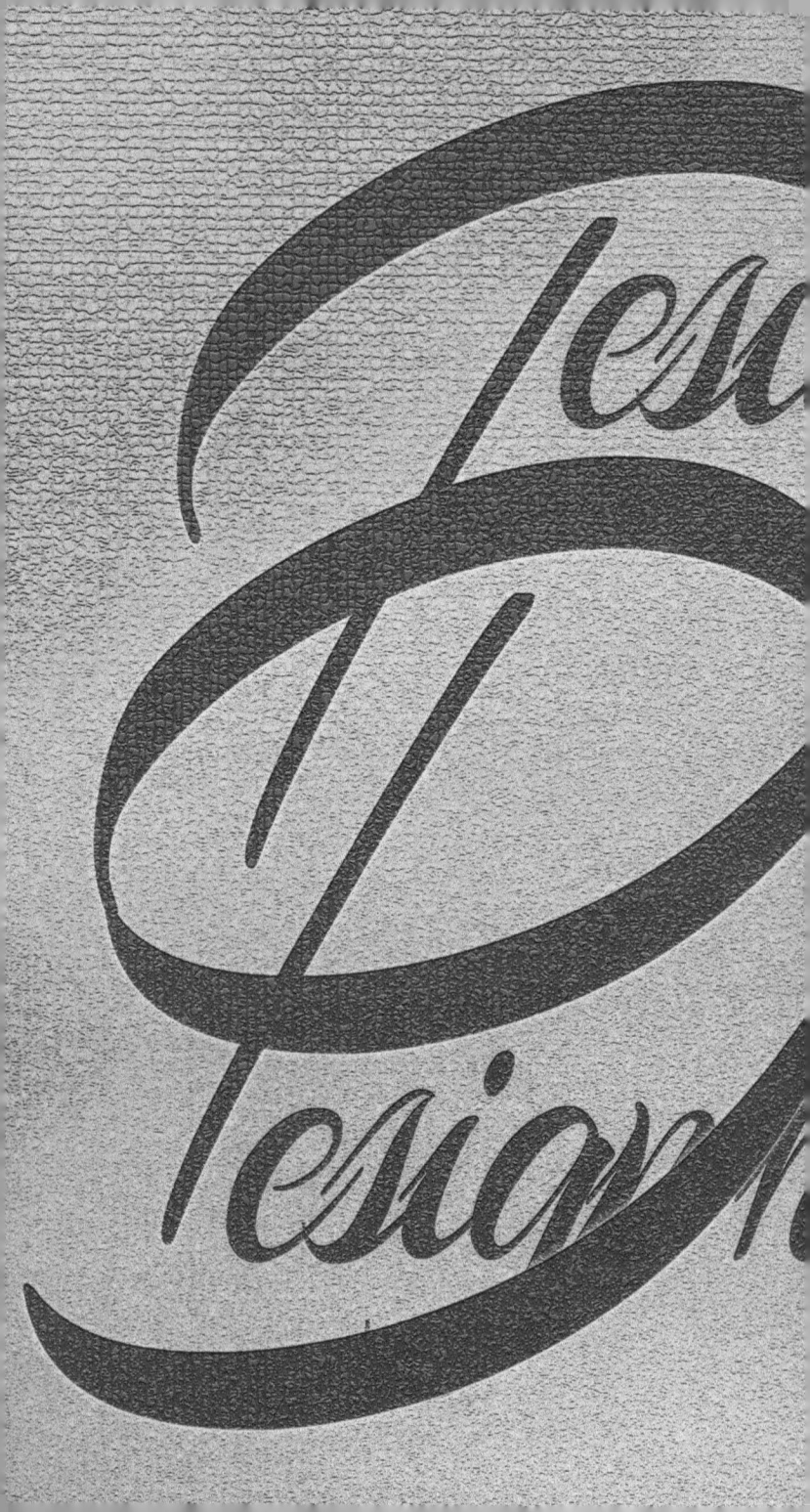

things?

Surely.

ppiness?

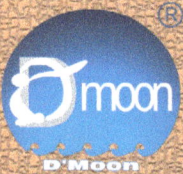

Credit goes to
author Astron Hues,
and the team of designers,
photographers, cartoonists,
and editors at the publisher: D'Moon

ISBN: 978-1-933187-13-6

Slight variations may occur
as part of the print-on-demand process
since each book is manufactured in its entirety.

Your feedback is most welcome ~
publisher@worldculturepictorial.com

Quest & Design...

AS YOU WISH

Astron Hues

d'moon books

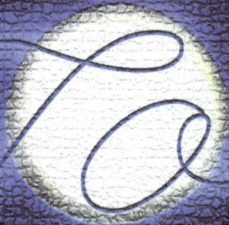

beloved

Preface

So much in life is design,
designed as desired.
Such as fashion,
architecture, sports teams,
and so on, so forth.

Design romantic dinners?
Sure, we can.
        Candlelight dinners
regularly popular.
Design true love?
Eh...

Design spacecrafts into space?
Surely, there are plenty:
Celestral Design of planets
Milky Way has been
a constant muse.

Fun to design,
Challenge to quest:
can Life be designed,
or redesigned
as all desire happiness?

Universe invites us
        into a new year
on the very generous Earth –
Lucky you, lucky me,
another youngest year
of mine, of yours, isn't it?

Join me!

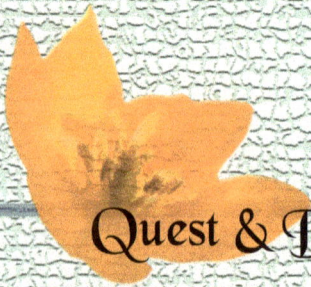

Quest & Design

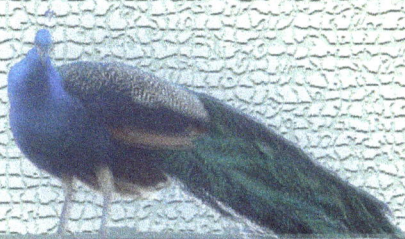

Quest & Design

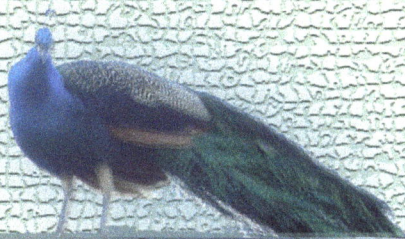

As You Wish

13

Quest & Design

Read more (Appendix)   64 - 71

◆Three Steps Wiser◆
- Reading and Reflection Vol. 03
released in 2018 (in full color)

◆Six Steps Wiser◆
- Reading and Reflection Vol. 06
released in 2021
designed art b&w interior print

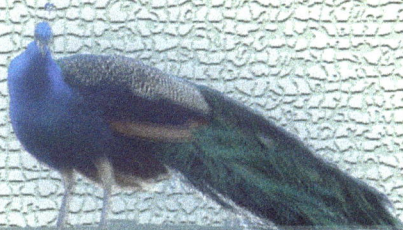

As You Wish

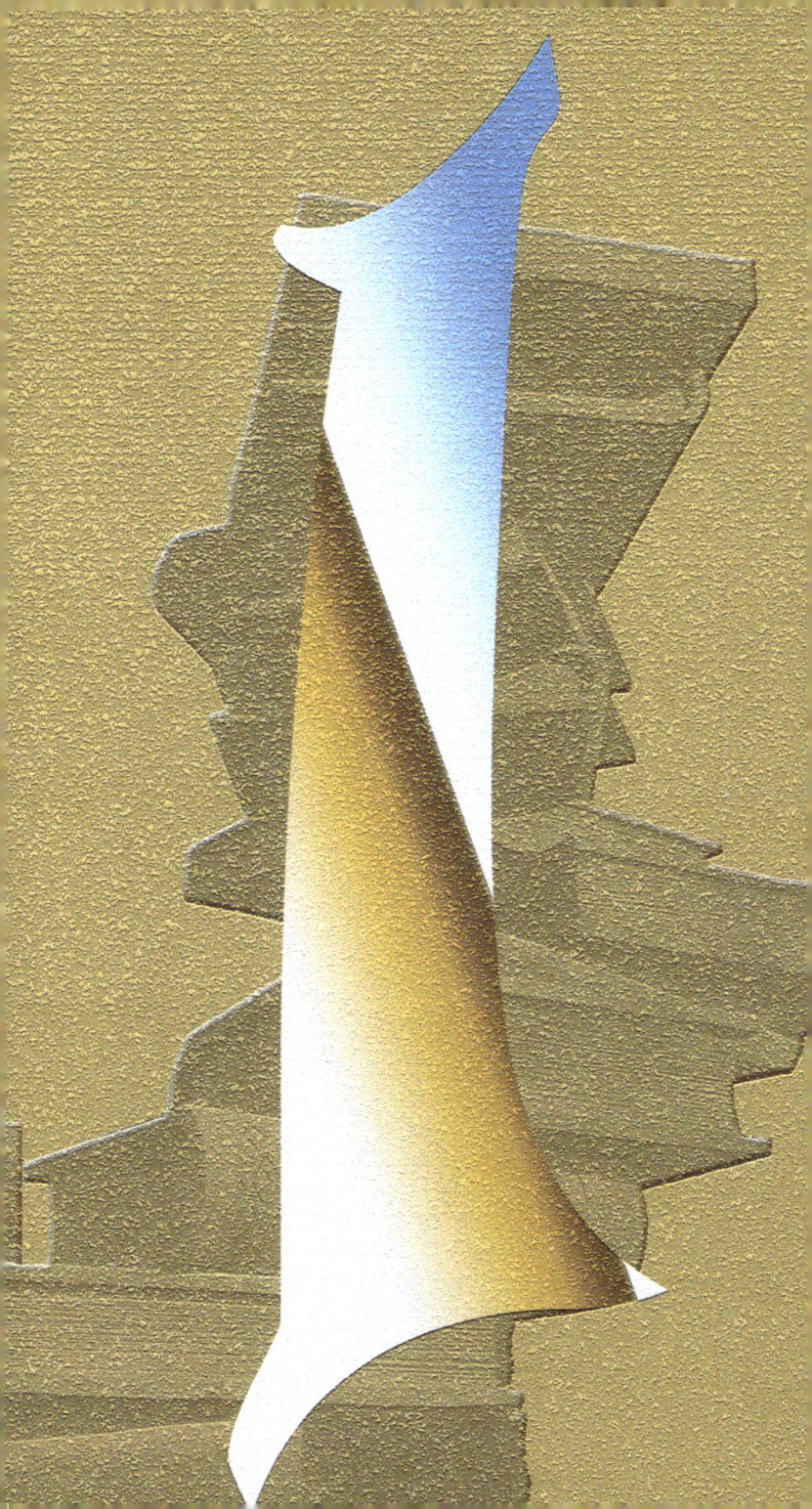

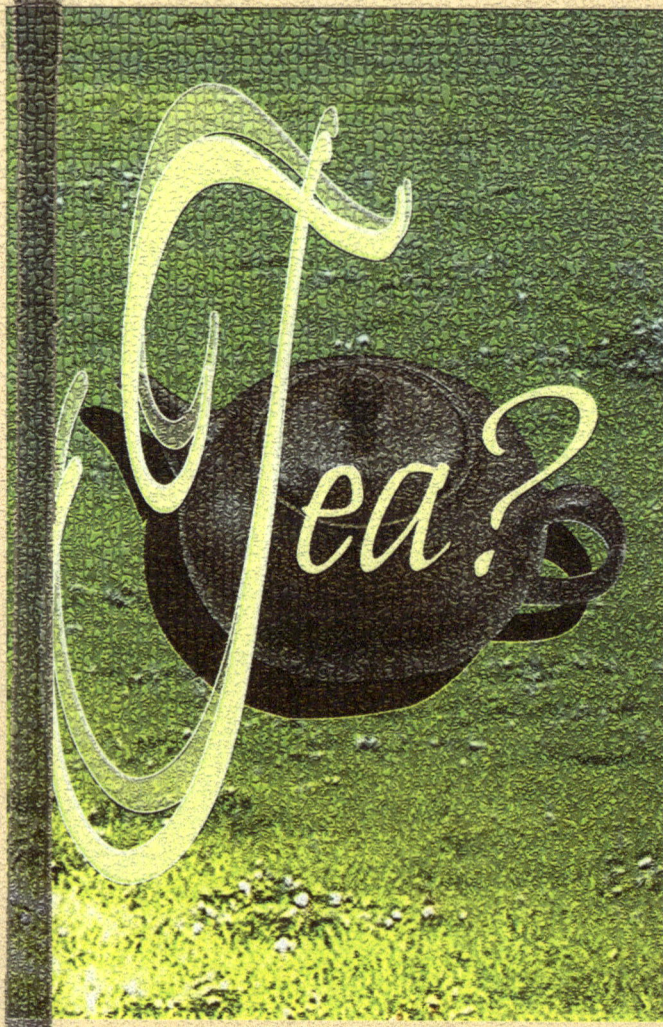

As You Wish

1. Wishing You Were Here

Morning,
Outside the window,
the sky is blue,
trees green.
Another beautiful day,
wishing you were here,
wishing we were
dining together.
The usual question,
very first, would be:
coffee or tea?
The usual votes
would go for green tea.

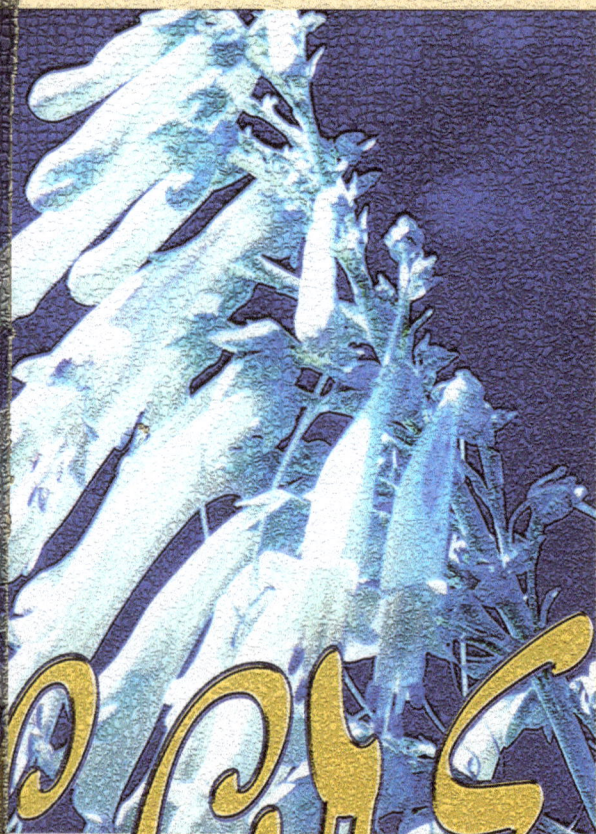

care

As You Wish

2. What can I do for you?

Miss those joyful moments.
Miss conversation over tea.
Miss chat over coffee
with or without dessert.
Miss jokes, laughter... That
"what can I do for you?"
never slips away from our
chat, each time we meet,
as it never slips away
from our hearts.
The care, so profound...
distance, stretching farther,
time of separation,
stretching longer.
Miss you all.

How are you?

3. Warm. Unequivocal.

Facemasks are
daily norm,
like runaways
from hospitals.
Have tried not
letting news surprise
or dispirit daily life.
"How are you"
means so much.
"Fine, and you"
means so much.
Much more than
an usual greeting.

Health Fortune

4. Fortune wears a hat

Folks encourage one another
to stay healthy.
Facemask a constant
patient messenger:
"unhealthy" is a word
unaffordable to be ignored.
Unhealthy? Terribly
unfortunate.
The tone of Fortune
is shifting
from dollar signs to state of
fitness.
Fortune is now
wearing a hat,
"Health" embroidered on it.

Thinking of you

As You Wish

5. Youngest Year

Just a few unturned pages
on the desk calendar,
waving goodbye
to the near past.
Yes, we are among
those lucky ones
invited to meet a new year.
Another youngest
    year of youth.
Another youngest
    year of middle age.
Another youn
    year of elderly.
Thinking of you!

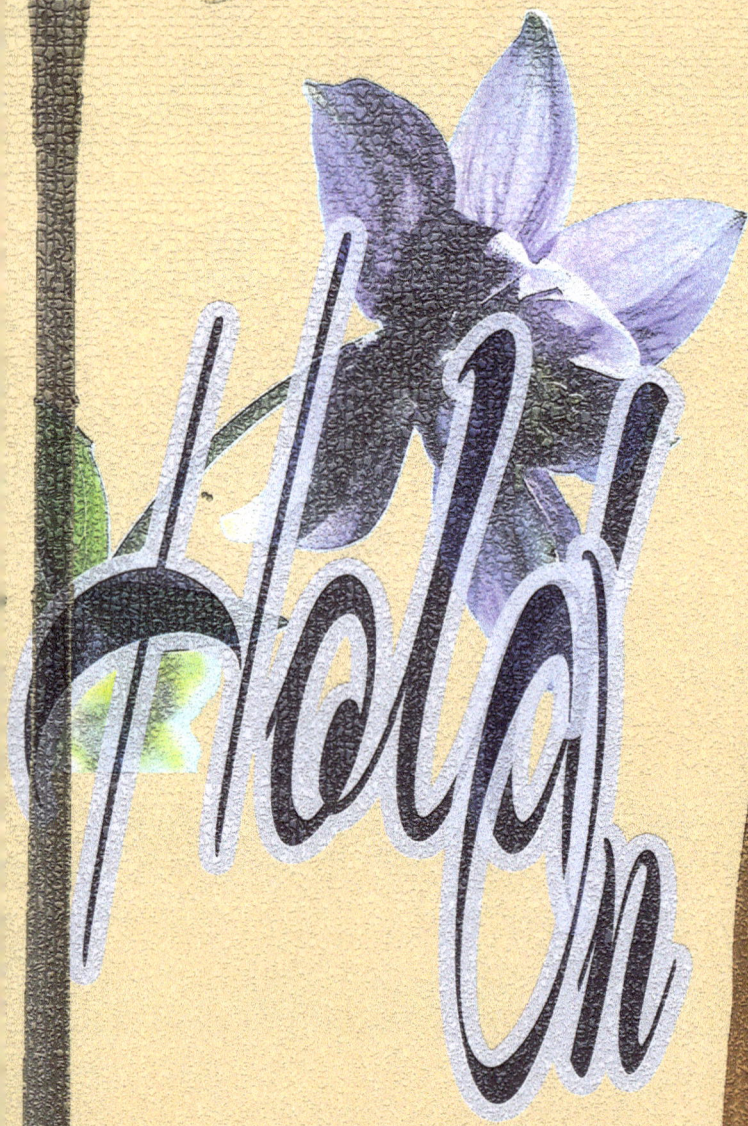

Quest & Design

Hold On

28

6. Slow down, possible?

The English ivy
next to my desk calendar takes
pride in non-stop growing.
The clock?
Non-stop ticking, ticking.
Time is flying away, non-stop.
And much faster. Although
no proof, nor learning tells me so.
Weekdays follow
weekends. End of month tails
beginning of each month.
Then, a new year,
waiting for nobody,
rings the bell.
Don't you feel the same way?

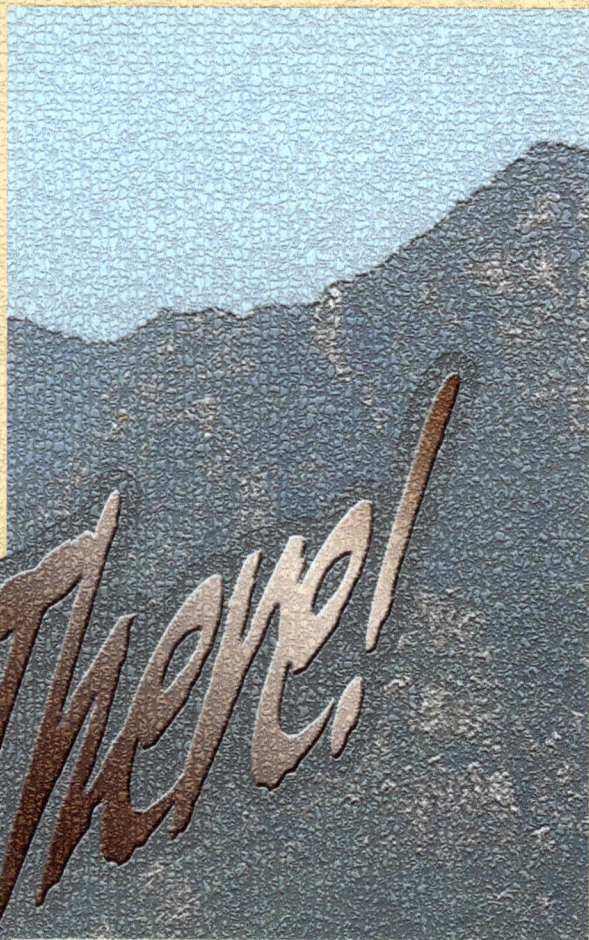

There!

As You Wish

7. Look up or look down?

Day in, day out,
most become busier.
Smartphones are
upgraded fast, updated faster,
and consequently
get much more attention
from nearly all.
Millions (perhaps billions)
feed, and read, the phones:
look at diners in restaurants,
pedestrians on sidewalks...
and at night before lights-out.
I guess those not bothered
by the rings would look around,
look up,
and enjoy
more, than those
heads down...

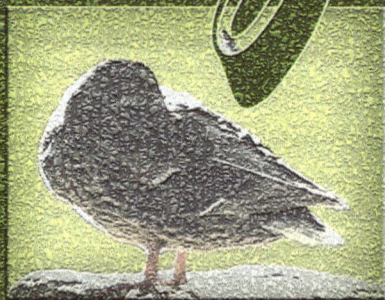

Quest & Design

Hey!

As You Wish

8. Future in Fashion of Haste

Day is rushing in
and Night rushing out.
More rush hours
in daily doings
rather than
rush hours in traffic.
Future joins
the fashion of haste,
like earnest runners
in competit
dashing
into present.

Quest & Design

Good Fluck

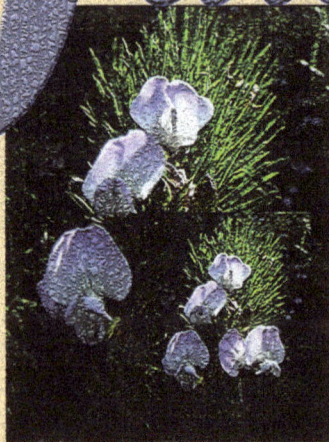

34

As You Wish

9. Check the Calendar

New year entering
the front door,
would check the desk calendar,
tear off page by page,
blow them quietly away,
disappearing into thin air...
Horizon at dawn.
What would ride winds
into life?
Wild guess?
No chance.

Common sense

As You Wish

10. Healthier, Merrier

As newly discovered,
Fortune is Health,
Health is Fortune.
Could Life be re-designed
to keep fit,
to keep our fortune?
Sounds simple.
The healthier, the merrier.
Makes sense.
Indeed.
Thinking of you!

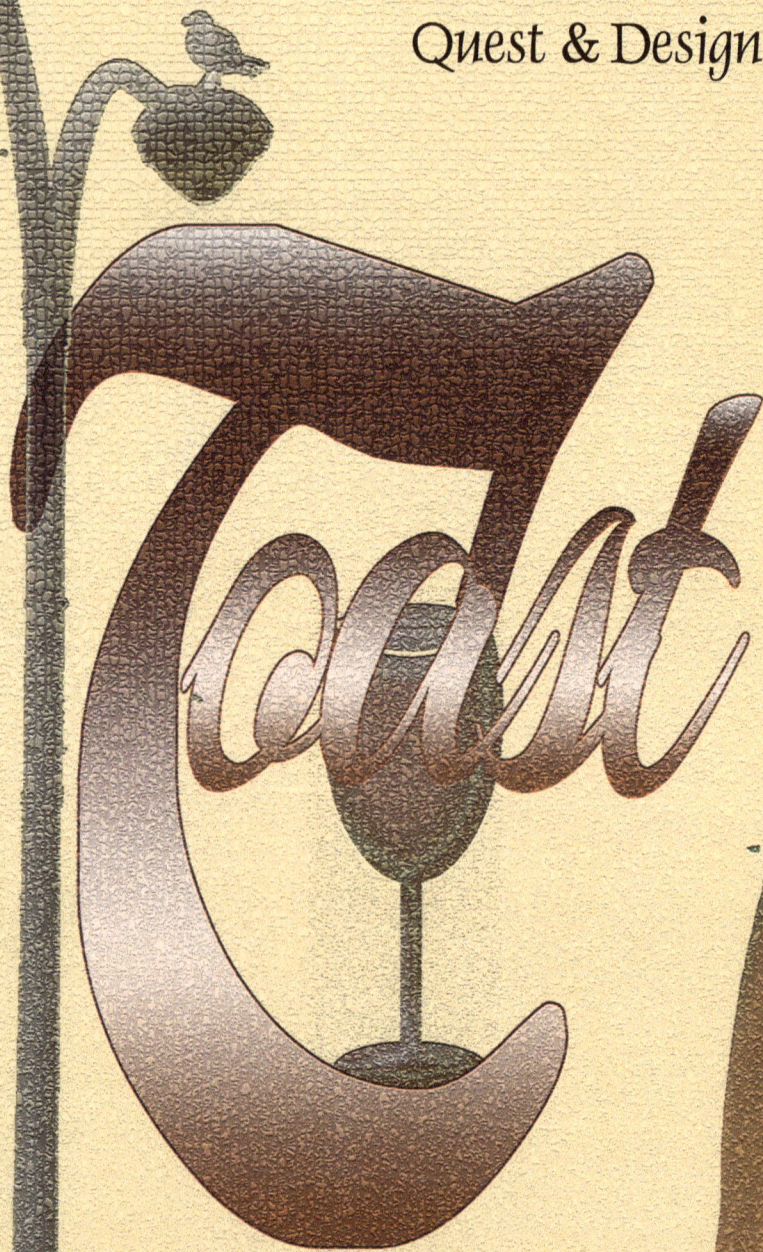

Toast

11. As You Wish

How to re-design Life?
And which way?
The merrier, the healthier.
What is riding winds
rushing in from horizon?
No one knows.
Only wish –
wish the best,
as I do, and,
with my whole heart,
wish the best for you,
as you wish.

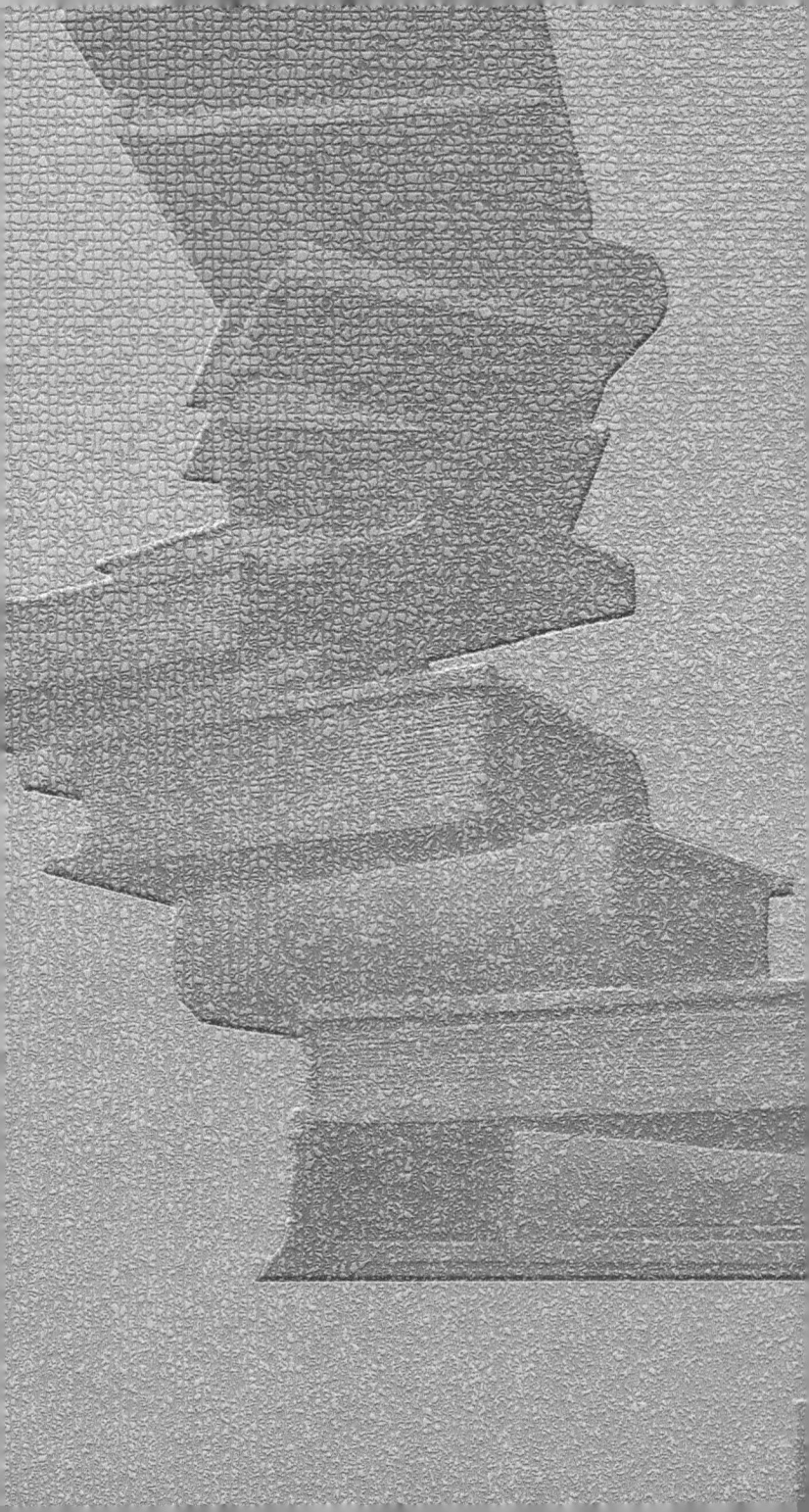

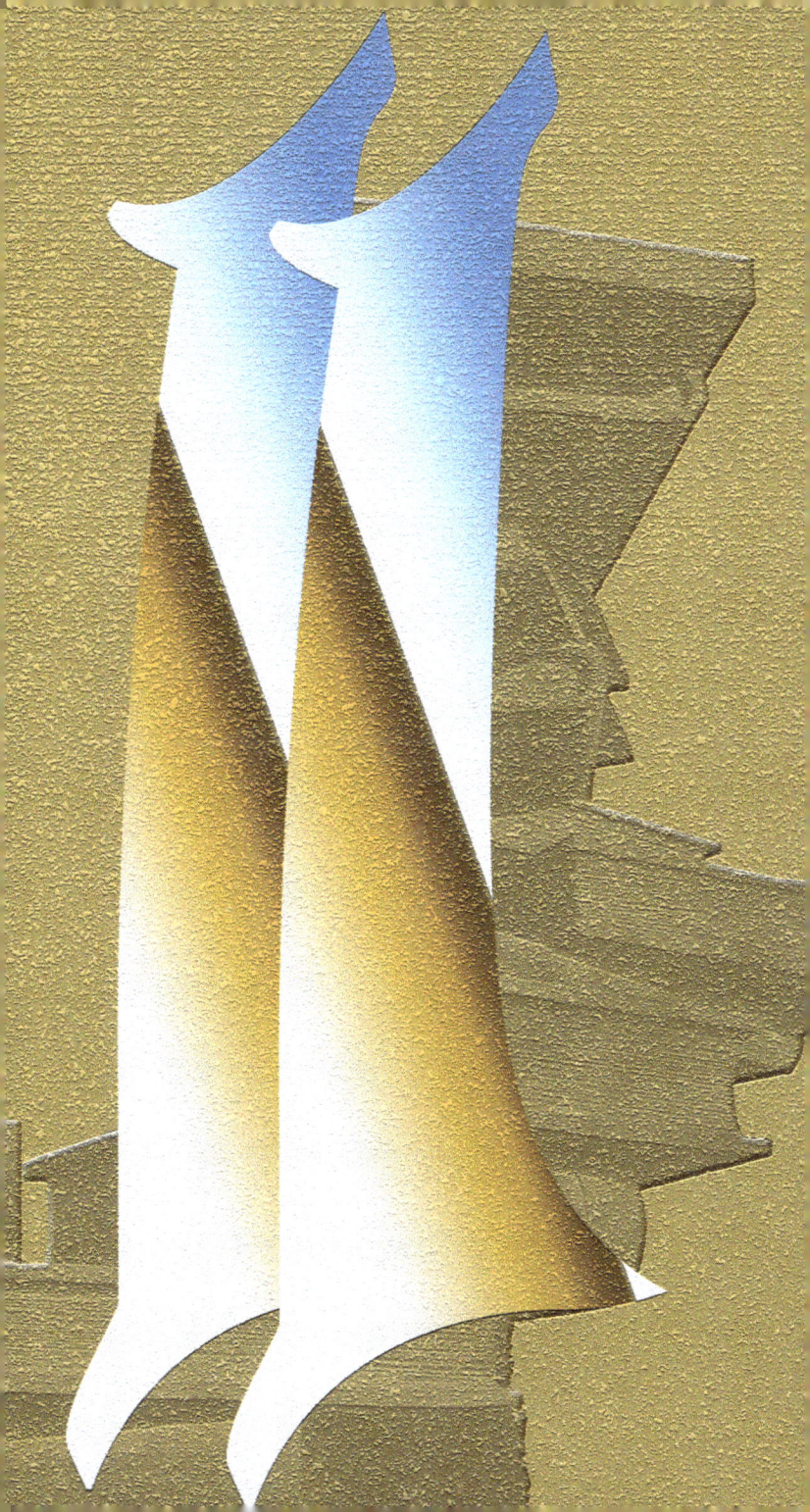

20-straight win 2002

As You Wish

Baseball, so much fun,
no wonder it's grown
so popular out of
child's play
as illustrated
in children's book
"A Little Pretty Pocket-Book"
by well-known John Newbery,
into serious sports
competition,
as in the movie Moneyball
(Brad Pitt as GM).

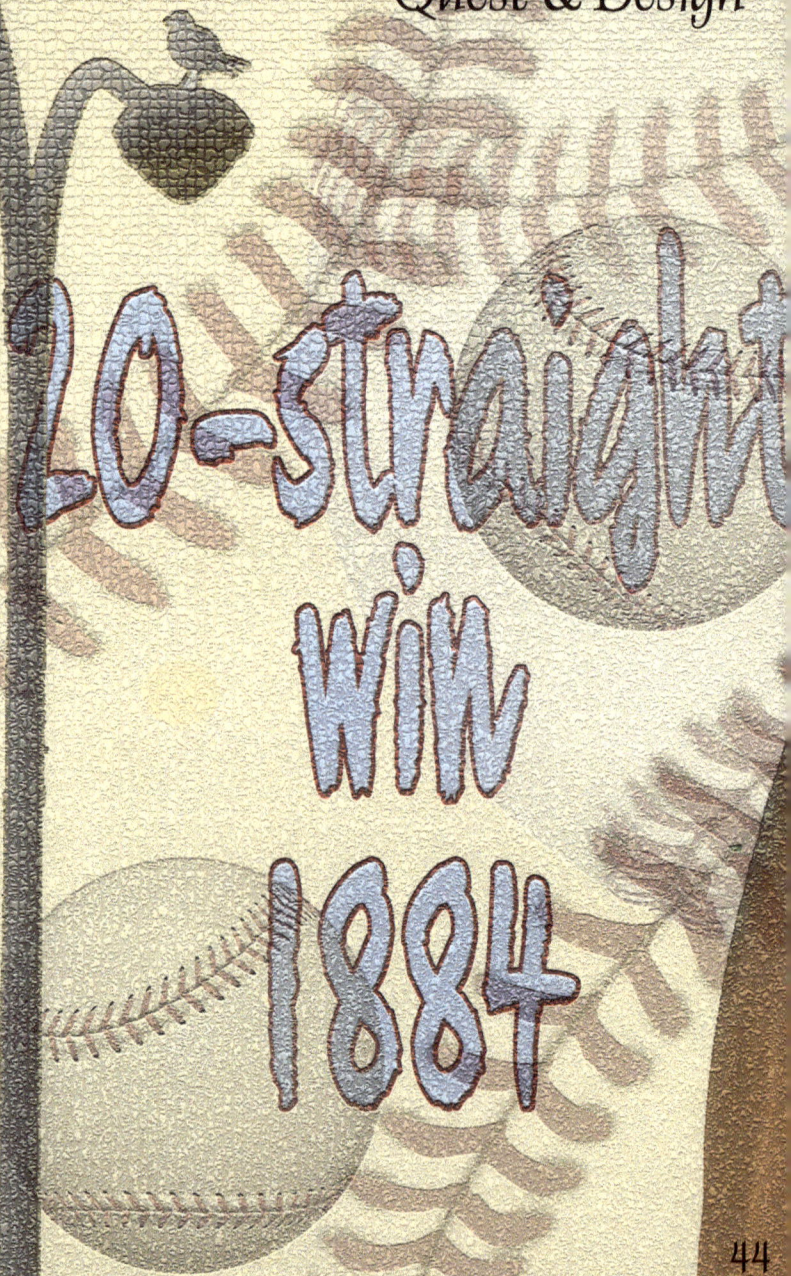

Quest & Design

20-straight
win
1884

44

As You Wish

Moneyball or not?
See what happened
in 1884
and what happened
in 2002 –
audience roaring
after the announcer's
anouncement in the movie,
and now,
spirit still soaring.
"Insane"? Oh no.

bat-and-ball game since 1740s

As You Wish

Like an
unchallenged king
since 1884,
the 20 wins in a row
sat there for 118 years,
until 2002!
The thrill, like thunder,
striking
audience off their seats,
roaring.
The winner is
Oakland Athletics.

118-year record

As You Wish

All baseball teams are
designed to win.
Big funds to sign on top players.
Who would disagree
that it is "moneyball"?

However, a 2002 straight
20-game win obviously
speaks otherwise,
a poor team
constrained by $38 million
against
a team
three times richer.

118th year: the A's ...

As You Wish

No money means
no top players.
hopelessness.
Slim chance
to stay in the game.
Moneyball, indeed.
If invisible money runs
the baseball field, there must
be something else
invisible
taking over the 2002
Oakland A's game.

all teams
designed
to win

As You Wish

Limited money.
2002 General Manager
Billy Beane
(portrayed by Brad Pitt
in "Moneyball")
hired "defective"
players.
Furthermore,
he traded two best
to put what is
in his vision
into the field.

what
crowns
the I winner?

As You Wish

Audience's "insane" excitement
is generated by a GM's
"insane" decision
which is incomprehensible,
impossible for any to agree.

Beane's decisions
astonishingly defy
baseball's "norm".
Yet, GM Beane
does not sway one bit
nor blink,
but firmly
unfolds the blueprint
in his mind.

2002 winner's money: $38 million

As You Wish

The intensity,
the sensation,
bursts out
when Oakland Athletics
wins 19 games in a row.
One more! One more!
One more win to break
the American League
consecutive-win
record,
established in 1884.

2002 winner's players: "written off"

As You Wish

(When backed by big money,
some would
confidently say,
certainly, why not?
Wish you could
as you wish.)

What makes Billy Beane
believe
under-appreciated athletes
will win?
Something invisible
inside him.
Intuition.
If not, what else?

2002 winner's team: "defective"

As You Wish

So, back to the quest –
all teams
are designed to win.
What crowns
the only winner?
If money's
not decisive
in 2002,
it must be
Beane's "intuition".

what, beyond "design"?

As You Wish

Teams can
be designed
for win,
A's 2002 GM
Billy Beane's
"intuition"?

Probably not.

Appendix

A
Read more

Appendix

d'mom books

Three Steps Wiser
Dear Goodluck

World
Culture
Pictorial
Reading &
Reflection
Vol 5

Read more

Six Steps Wiser

Dave Goodluck

World
Culture
Pictorial
Reading &
Reflection
Vol. 6

Appendix

Book of L

ISBN 978-1-933187-90-7

90000

9 781933 187907

Read more

BOOK OF L

Quotable Wit & Wisdom

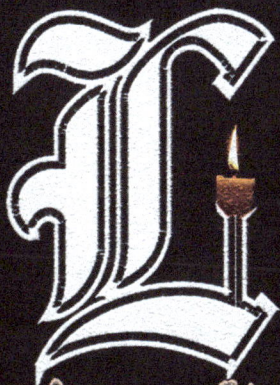

Dr. Common Sense

dimoon books

Appendix

Read more

time travelers Who isn't? — Lu Queen